VENUS
SENIOR

Is Your *Cash* in Your *Doctor's Stash?*

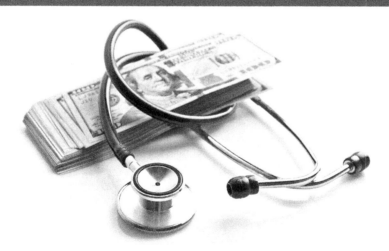

9 Ways to Find Money and Pay Less on Medical Bills

ISBN: 978-1-948777-20-9

DISCLAIMER

The information I share in this book is based on my twenty-three years of personal experience with many account issues and patient inquires that I had the pleasure to resolve. This book is not intended to harm or discredit any provider, doctor, or their billing staff. This information is simply being provided to help patients navigate the medical billing system to help them to save money, find money, and pay less on medical expenses.

ACKNOWLEDGMENTS

Thank you, God!

Thank you for giving me the understanding and gift to serve both the patient and the provider.

Thank you to everyone who pushed me and assisted with the completion of this project!

I thank my past, current, and future state of experience to the medical billing revenue cycle, which sparked a passion in me to help "everyone to get understanding."

Special thanks for your pre-orders and patience.

Tarsha Burley

Velma Lewis

Ziyadah Joynes

Cynthia Middleton

Kim Brown

DEDICATION

Dear Reader,

I hope this book will inspire those of you who work in and out of the health care community. I believe the information offered will empower you to seek a deeper understanding of your healthcare benefits and outstanding medical bills. With this new knowledge, individuals and families can transform their financial circumstances. The freedom offered from a surprise credit can be applied to other bills or extra shoes for the child who won't stop growing. Or even a trip!

At times, trips seem impossible because the complexity of a patient's unexpected financial responsibility is difficult to navigate. You need an advocate. You want an advocate. Feel free to reach out to me at info@ allaspectsmedical.com. I promise you: no question is too big. I have compassion and empathy for the resolution of your medical billing issues. More often than not, patients are faced with the thought of being kicked out of a facility during their end of life care because of the lack understanding of coverage and/or ability to pay. This is ridiculous. This has to stop. This is absurd. I don't want this to happen to you. I speak from experience.

I dedicate this book to two very special people who experienced the insurance and provider potholes as they transitioned into their afterlife, and to all who will read it and are able to take action.

The first of these two people is my dad. On March 14, 2019, my dad, Johnny Boy, went into the hospital. He had been diagnosed with a mass in his prostate and lesions on his bones. It was cancer. During his second week in the hospital, he decided he wanted hospice care.

The hospice social workers stated that it would be difficult to find a facility that would a) take his insurance and b) have an available bed. Furthermore, according to them, it would be difficult to determine the percentage of his income that would be used to take care of excess costs outside of his insurance because he received SSDI and Medicaid.

It was initially stated that due to the type of coverage he had, he could not be transferred to a facility in the state in which he was currently receiving his care. On the fifteenth day into his transition, it was stated hospice would be done right in the hospital where he was receiving care. In a matter of minutes, my heart, my love, my everything right after Christ, took his last breath. I was right beside him, holding his hand.

It ended with the treating facility being paid roughly $60,000, which included charges for medications that my father refused but were still reflected on the bill.

Next is my aunt, Sherrie Berrie. What I absolutely loved about her is that when she began to tap into the information that I shared with her regarding her healthcare treatment and coverage, she listened and began to take action. She was diagnosed with the most aggressive and rare form of stage 4 metastatic breast cancer, and she needed to make sure that she was covered by insurance.

Her journey with insurance involved learning how to reach out to her providers and insurance carrier to find out what was covered and what was not. She learned that she needed to advocate for herself by asking questions to the insurance company, the provider, and two different breast cancer community programs.

My aunt told me that the information I provided ensured that she understood what she could do to maintain her team of providers (PCP, oncologist, and her surgeon), and she was so glad that she began to participate in recording videos and engage in conversations about the details regarding insurance coverage. Her battle was short, but in that short time, she took action that enabled her to get the coverage she needed.

However, it was not enough; during her illness she was denied care from fourteen different facilities. Finally, she was transferred between five different facilities within her two-week transition to the end of her earthly life. Her fourth transfer only lasted five days. When the money ran out, we had to look for another facility. Thankfully, the fifth and final transfer was to a not-for-profit facility that offered a beautiful, heaven-like experience. This Christian hospice facility didn't require payment upon her entrance, and they provided my aunt with the best level of care.

She received her wings on March 14, 2020.

Learn from these short, medical billing end-of-life experiences to get an understanding of your healthcare benefits, out-of-pocket expenses, medical bills, and what financial impact it can have on your family and your community. If it is within your control, choose your insurance carrier, providers and facilities wisely, and—most importantly—read your explanation of benefits before you pay.

Venus "Patient Account Detective" Senior

CRCS-P CRCS-I

Member of American Association of Healthcare Administration Management (AAHAM)

FOREWORD

For me and so many others, paying a visit to the doctor's office while having the ability to pull out my insurance card gave me a sense of comfort and security. I knew that I was covered. But while that is important to know, having a full understanding of how your copayments are applied and whether or not you have any outstanding credits is equally important. If you ever decide to do some research, you'll probably be surprised to learn the amount of credits you have in your account.

What I like about Venus and her book is her level of compassion and concern to make sure the readers are aware of the importance of understanding your health insurance and how you can save and find money. In Chapter 3, Venus takes a deeper dive into explaining what you should do when you learn of credits sitting on your account. So many people are taken advantage of due to the lack of knowledge; however; this book is a page-turner full of secrets related to your out-of-pocket expenses, which the health industry fails to disclose. Thank you, Venus, for educating our community and providing me with a new sense of awareness that will help me and my family protect our cash from our doctor's stash!

Z Joynes

TABLE OF CONTENTS

Disclaimer iii

Acknowledgments iv

Dedication v

Foreword ix

Introduction 1

Chapter 1: Is Your Cash in Your Doctor's Stash? 7

Chapter 2: Whose Bill Is It? 13

Chapter 3: Did You Overpay? 23

Chapter 4: Do You Have Multiple Carriers? 31

Chapter 5: Do You Know the Difference Between
Medicare and Medicaid? 35

Chapter 6: Pay Less for Medical Expenses Before and After Service .. 41

Chapter 7: How Does COVID-19 Impact Your Medical Bills? 57

Chapter 8: What Should You Remember When Using a Flexible
Spending Account (FSA) Card or a Health Savings Account (HSA)
Card? 61

Chapter 9: Get Your Cash From Your Doctor's Stash 65

Appendix 1: Tips to Help You Get Your Money Back 71

Appendix 2: Key Terms 76

Appendix 3: Testimonials 83

Appendix 4: Important Websites 86

INTRODUCTION

Wisdom is the principal thing; therefore get wisdom. And in all your getting, get understanding.

Proverbs 4:7 (New King James Version)

Here to Help You

I solve problems with bills. I am a billing angel. I am an EOB translator. I will go right up the chain and communicate for you on your behalf. I have a heart to help patients, people just like you, who receive surprise medical bills or bills that are incorrect.

I want to fix the system—one bill at a time, one patient at a time. But I didn't always know that was my gift. I have always liked to look at numbers and compare them to what was reflected on the patient's account. I have been told that I could help doctors with their denials, but I really wanted to help patients receive the correct bill and understand it. I once got a patient a refund for $749.69, even though she had been waiting three months for her credit. Many of us are not even aware that a credit exists. But we absolutely know that bills exist.

Sometimes we have a tendency to sit on bills that we don't know how to pay; when money is tight, we might put the bills aside. We might not even want to look at another bill because we think, *Here's another financial obligation that I simply don't have the money to pay,* or, *I don't understand why I am being billed for something I thought my insurance took care of or told me would be covered.*

You might have bills you are sitting with right now, bills you're not sure what to do with. I can help you. These bills are taking up your energy and time and taking up space on your table. Let me help you clear them. I took accounting courses, and I was blessed to land a job at the Georgetown Lombardi Comprehensive Cancer Center. I got a sense of what the patients were going through. They came to the front desk, and they could not get definitive answers regarding their bills. They were sometimes brushed off because the front desk representative could not explain the details of the bill. That frustrated me because the front desk staff should be somewhat familiar with benefits, and/or be able to explain the details of the bill, and/or direct the patient to the insurance company for clarification.

After the assignment with the Lombardi Cancer Center, I was then assigned to the unified billing office for Georgetown physicians. I had some knowledge about how to help patients, but I didn't know everything I needed to know in order to help everyone. But in that office, two decades ago, I met a woman by the name of Cynthia Middleton who showed me how to navigate the billing system and gave me a crash course on Healthcare Billing 101. I was intrigued. We were posting payments received by the payer, patient, insurance company, or another party. We were interpreting invoices from the insurance company. We saw many errors on patient accounts. One such example included patients being billed for amounts that should have been applied as an adjustment per their insurance EOB.

I was diligent in wanting to do this job correctly. I aced it, developed a passion for it, and then wanted to train others to do the same. As I started to train others, I realized that some people were not passionate about the job. I wanted patients' concerns heard and their inquiries resolved. This is very important because as staff of the medical billing office, we ultimately determine the fate of what patients are being billed for. Money was not being posted correctly, and patients were being charged for amounts that they did not owe. This did not sit right with me because it meant we sometimes collected money that was not owed to the provider. While we sorted that out, that same cash built up and grew interest in the doctor's stash.

I had to explain bills to patients when they did not understand them. And like you, they found that bills were sometimes really confusing. I could look at the EOB and help them. My gift was to assist people who were in despair of understanding and paying their bills. I wanted to help people who had been wronged. I want to make things right for them. If this is you, keeping reading, because this book is for you.

I have worked for several healthcare organizations in areas such as registration, follow-up, customer service, Medicare billing, cash posting, financial counseling, and management. I saw that staff and management sometimes did not know how to navigate or did not even understand the billing system. I knew that I needed to make a change. I became that person who took the time to train and teach individuals everything that I knew. I took certification classes to ensure that I was current on laws, rules, and regulations, so that as a professional healthcare revenue cycle leader, my team and I complied with those laws, and we operated with integrity as it related to healthcare billing and the patient experience.

I know that healthcare and insurance industries can be very complex if patients do not understand their benefits, the revenue cycle, or their responsibilities. I believe that if employers would take the time to provide benefit education, then patients would understand their benefits. This would help patients save money and understand how to pay less on their medical expenses. This understanding will increase your peace of mind and your bank account.

What You Understand, You Get to Keep!

Navigating the system between the doctor's office and the insurance company is important. Often, misunderstandings occur between these two systems. Either entity might drop the ball. But I can help you with that navigation. Help you build understanding. The insurance company will help you. Do not be afraid. Be courageous, and reach out. Document those calls each time. Remember to ask for a reference number for each call. As "The Patient Account Detective," I, Venus Senior, intend to share how to pay less on healthcare and medical expenses and help you find money due back to you from healthcare providers.

I want to acknowledge that sometimes doctors don't even understand how the billing system works. They are concerned with treating the patient. But when the doctor becomes a patient, he or she is surprised by the complexity of the system. One such doctor said to me: "Why didn't anyone tell me I would get two bills after my emergency room visit? I paid my ER copay! I would never do this to my patients, and I am a doctor. I will make sure my patients are informed."

Let me help you stay informed. Patients get care; providers get paid; and everyone can get understanding.

In the following chapters you will learn the secrets to:

- Finding your cash/credit that is temporarily being held in the doctor's stash.

- Paying less on medical expenses.

- Requesting a refund that can be used to pay past, current, or future medical expenses.

- Understanding specific aspects of your benefits.

- Knowing whether or not you are being billed correctly.

NOTES

1

IS YOUR CASH IN YOUR DOCTOR'S STASH?

Did you know that you, the insurance company, and a third party could all inadvertently pay the same bill to the doctor's office? Has this happened to you? And when that happened, where did that money go? Did it go to an account and earn interest? Who is going to get that earned interest? Do you know how to check your doctor's stash for your cash?

A "doctor's stash" is a bank account that accumulates payments remitted by patients, insurance companies, and other parties not owed to the doctor (provider). The money sits in the doctor's bank account and collects interest. This is also true for facilities and healthcare organizations.

There are several reasons why patients have cash in their doctor's stash and are entitled to a refund. For example:

- Overpayment has occurred, which includes any payment paid by any party over the charged amount.

7

- Payments have been paid upfront, and then the insurance company made a payment.
- Proper adjustment has not been applied.
- Duplicate billing has occurred.
- The patient has paid the wrong doctor or provider.

In subsequent chapters, I delve into these examples in detail. However, in this chapter, I want to cover one of the most problematic examples. In some cases, the provider or facility may not tell a patient that there is a credit on their account. The provider continues to request or require payment for services rendered, or for prepayment of future services. Often copays, deductibles, coinsurance, and other amounts are paid upfront because the doctor/hospital requests or requires it before services are rendered. This happens daily in facilities across the country.

How does the hospital determine the amount to be paid in advance? First, with the patient's insurance information, the hospital runs a verification of benefits, and then they can determine the estimated amount that the patient has to pay upfront. This is often the deductible. The deductible can be applied to the first bill processed and could also include copay, coinsurance, and non-covered charges.

If a patient pays the hospital the stated deductible amount, and then after the services are rendered, the doctors involved in the care a) bill their claims, and b) the hospital bills their claims, unintentional confusion can occur. The patient will not know which bill the deductible has been applied to until they receive their Explanation of Benefits (EOB) or contact their insurance. The deductible amount could be applied to the doctor's bill first, or it could be applied to the hospital bill first. There is no way to know before the procedure or during registration which claim will be processed first and applied to the deductible.

If the doctor's claim is processed first, then the doctor can bill the patient for the total or a portion of the deductible amount that the patient has already paid to the hospital. I know this sounds confusing. You, dear patient, were asked to pay at the hospital—and now you got a second bill? If the hospital bill is processed first, then the amount that the patient paid before the procedure stays with the hospital.

All of this will surely confuse the patient. The patient's deductible responsibility depends on which claim has been processed first. So when there is confusion, you, dear reader, can ask:

Which Claim Has Been Processed First?

You might have to call the hospital to request a refund. When doing so, please remember that the hospital may deduct any copays and/ or coinsurance amounts out of the larger amount you paid up front, and then issue a refund. If you paid the hospital $1,000, and there is a copay of $50, and a coinsurance of $150, then your refund will be $800. I understand you might feel awkward calling the hospital to ask for a refund, but remember that money belongs to you. If you don't call, your $800 grows interest in the hospital's stash.

When there is extra cash (overpayment made by a patient or an other party) reflected as a credit balance on a patient's account, refunds are owed back to the patient, or the insurance company, or a third party (workers' compensation, auto insurance, law office). This credit balance can be from services rendered recently, or from several years ago. A credit balance does not expire. If you don't ask about the credit and then claim it, physicians may or may not tell you that the credit exists. It is still sitting there, growing interest. I have witnessed credits on patients' accounts for services rendered as far back as seventeen years ago.

By now you must be wondering if you have a credit with your physician or hospital. But perhaps you are not sure how to ask if you have this credit. Keep reading! I want you to have your refund. I want you to get your cash. The following eight chapters will tell you how to determine if you have a credit, who to ask if you have one, how to pay less on your medical bills, and how to get your cash back.

TAKEAWAYS:

- Always ask the provider if your account reflects a credit that should be refunded or transferred to an outstanding balance that you may have.
- Make sure when making payments that you are paying the correct provider.
- Deductibles will be applied to the claim that has been processed first by the insurance carrier.

KEY TERMS:

Co-insurance

An out-of-pocket expense: a percentage of the cost for the service that was rendered that the patient is required to pay. Percentages can run from 10%–30%, and in some cases more. For example, if the coinsurance amount is 10% and the cost of service is $1,000, the patient's payment responsibility is $100.

Copay

A flat fee paid for certain covered services, such as doctor visits, emergency room visits, prescriptions, or in-patient visits.

Deductible

An amount required to be paid by the patient each year before the healthcare plan starts paying benefits.

Doctor's Stash

Overpayments remitted to providers from insurance companies and patients, or other parties that sit in their bank account or on their books and collect interest.

Overpayment

Payment made in excess of what is or was due.

NOTES

2

WHOSE BILL IS IT?

Frances Turner, forty-seven, has no preexisting health conditions and works as a sales associate for a marketing company that requires her to travel in multiple states. Though she lives in California, she received a bill from a medical facility in Washington, DC, where she has never traveled. She called the medical facility to inquire why she was receiving a bill. After reviewing her account, it was confirmed that she never went to that facility nor had she received any of the services stated on the bill.

After their review, the facility agreed to her dispute and removed all charges. It was later revealed to Frances that her information was included in the file due to a typographical error. There were multiple patients with the same name (multiple Turners born on the same day but in different years), and her name had been added to that file. The medical facility advised her that somehow her information was provided, but they did not have any valid IDs or signatures on file to validate that she was responsible for the charges. Unfortunately, she was not provided any additional details as to how the facility acquired her information.

If this happens to you—and statistically, it probably will—you will want to a) review your bill, b) review the location of services, c) review the date of birth, d) review the phone number and address, e) call the provider and ask them to review the bill, f) document the date and time of the call and who you spoke to, g) follow up one week later, and, h) if after a month, you have not received a resolution, feel free to email me at info@allaspectsmedical.com.

This Happens More Often Than You Think

In 2018, the population of America was roughly 327 million people. How many people do you think were surprised or caught off guard by a medical bill?

Over 186,504,000 people received a bill that did not belong to them.

Maybe you are one of these people. I want to help you solve this problem and help you help your friends and family with this same issue. I want to help the staff who work in doctor's offices who may not know that they are making mistakes.

Patients are sometimes billed for other patients' services because the billing staff may have selected the incorrect patient during registration. In 2018, a survey by the National Opinion Research Center (NORC. org) of the University of Chicago revealed that "57% of Americans have been surprised by a medical bill" that turned out not to be theirs. The surprise has multiple impacts: 1) The patient has been charged a $50 copay when, in fact, they don't owe one, and they don't know how to ask for that refund; 2) The doctor's office has received that copay and posted it to another patient's account, and is sometimes surprised to have to return it; 3) Interest may have grown on that $50 copay, and the return opens up the door for many questions with multiple parties. Doctors

14

may not know these errors are occurring, and many of these mistakes are completely unintentional.

So what can you do on your end when a surprise bill comes in the mail?

Review the EOB/bill carefully before making a payment.

When receiving the bill, review it in its entirety and verify that the following information is correct:

- Name on the bill (first, middle, and last)
- Date of birth
- Social Security Number
- Your address
- Your phone number
- The service date
- The service
- Insurance information

Before paying any bill received from a healthcare provider, compare the bill to the EOB to ensure that you are being billed and paying the correct amount.

What in the EOB Is This?

The EOB explains what the patient does and does not owe the provider.

The EOB is sent to the patient by the insurance company.

Although EOB statements are generally correct, providers may bill patients for services that the insurance company has stated are not the patient's responsibility. For example:

- Adjustments

- Non-covered services

- Services rendered with no waivers on file

- Past timely filing charges (charges that the provider did not bill in a timely manner)

Reviewing the EOB carefully is very important to make sure you are:

- Only paying the provider what is owed after benefits have been applied

- Not being billed for something the insurance carrier stated is not owed by the patient

- Not being billed for a service when the insurance carrier has requested additional information from the provider or the patient

There are instances where the provider would bill the insurance for a service, and the insurance would reply: *We request additional information. We need medical records in order to complete the processing of the claim.* The provider will then, in some cases, send the bill to you. When insurance requests for additional information from the provider, the provider cannot bill you. They have to send the requested information first so that the insurance carrier can complete the processing of the claim. This is one reason it is important to review your EOB before you pay anything.

Below is an example of an EOB statement from an insurance carrier. Pay attention to the following: amount billed, total charges billed to the carrier, discount amount, amount the provider should write off, the amount you owe, and finally where the service was rendered.

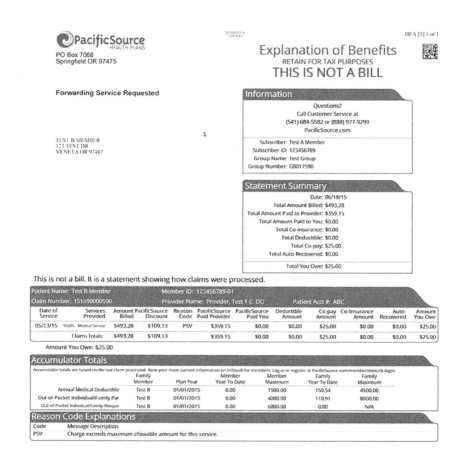

Was the Service Coded Correctly?

Healthcare providers and/or hospitals identify medical services with codes. Most patients do not notice these codes on their EOB, let alone understand what they mean. It is important to understand the meaning of these codes to ensure the billing reflects the correct services. I often tell patients to search for the CPT code on Google to get the exact description of a treatment or service they received. Certain service codes determine *out-of-pocket* expenses for the patient, for example, *preventative* versus *office* visits.

You may have selected a particular health insurance benefit level, and this level determines if preventative visits do or do not have "out-of-pocket" expenses. However, if you have been seen by a provider for a preventative visit, but by accident, it is coded as an office visit, then a charge for an "out-of-pocket" expense may appear on the bill. The exact amount of an "out-of-pocket expense" varies, and it could consist of a deductible, coinsurance, and/or a copay amount.

Additionally, there are three main medical service code types assigned by physicians: Procedure Code (CPT), Level, and Diagnoses (ICD-10). We will focus on procedure and diagnosis codes.

Procedure Code

Current procedural code terminology. Medical classification used to identity treatment.

Diagnosis Code

Describes diseases, illnesses, and injuries.

On the example EOB, you will only see the procedure code. The diagnosis code is located on the claim that went to the insurance carrier. When reviewing the EOB, pay the most attention to the CPT code. If you need information regarding the Dx submitted to the insurance carrier, pick up the phone and call them.

As you are reviewing the EOB, the following action steps may help you:

Step 1: Review the CPT code. (See above example: EOB 99205 - medical   service.)*

Step 2: Ask yourself if you had this service.

Step 3: Review the code to make sure the description matches the service.

*Google the following question: What does CPT code 99205 stand for? Remember to insert your particular CPT code in Google's search bar. I am using the number from the EOB sample above in order to show you the method. In other words, your search might look like this:

What does CPT code (fill in your number from your EOB) stand for?

Step 4: Call the billing office and ask them to review the charge, code, and chart to verify if you were billed correctly. You can tell them that you used Google to find your CPT code and have questions about how it aligns with the service you received.

Sometimes you may set up a regular preventative visit, and yet when you review your EOB, you are surprised to find that the visit contains two codes, or that the visit was coded as an office visit. Yet you know that you came in for a preventative visit. Preventative visits and office visits are not represented by the same code. Take Sally, for example:

Sally went to her healthcare provider for a preventative visit, which is free based on her health insurance benefit coverage. During the visit, the provider asked if she had any other health concerns she wanted to discuss. Sally told the provider about the pain in her back that she was experiencing. After discussing the issue with Sally, the provider prescribed muscle relaxers. When Sally received her medical bill—and also reviewed her EOB *before paying anything*—she noticed a charge for an "office visit" instead of a "preventative visit."

Sally called the healthcare provider's billing department and disputed the bill. She explained that her visit with the provider was preventative. She also shared that the provider asked if she had other concerns but did not inform her that by answering the question and receiving a prescription, it would result in a charge for an office visit, which then resulted in an out-of-pocket expense. The provider agreed to her dispute because he did not inform her of the additional charge and corrected the service code and billing. The bill was resubmitted to the insurance company and reprocessed and left Sally with no patient responsibility.

How to Notice a Duplicate Charge

When you've reviewed your bills in the past, have you ever wondered if you were being charged for a service twice? This can happen. Reviewing each charge and each line item on medical bills received from a healthcare provider is essential in order to make sure that there are no duplicate charges.

Example A: Two Duplicate Types of Strep Tests

Wanda went to her doctor's office due to a sore throat. Her doctor used one swab to test the back of her throat for strep. When Wanda received her bill, she noticed the following charges:

1. Strep A $120

2. Strep B $125

3. Strep A $120

Wanda's bill was incorrect because she was charged twice for the same strep test (#1 and #3).

Some services may look like duplicate charges but are not.

Example B: Not a Duplicate: Two Different Types of Strep Tests

Henry went to his doctor's office due to a sore throat. His provider used one swab to test the back of Henry's throat. When Henry received his bill, he noticed the following charges.

1. Strep A $120

2. Strep B $120

Henry's bill is correct because he was charged for two different types of strep tests, even though his throat was only swabbed once.

TAKEAWAYS:

- Review bills in their entirety and contact the provider's billing office for clarity on any questionable charge(s).
- Request immediate correction and removal of duplicate charge(s), and acquire the original or a copy of the EOB and your bill for your records. Also be sure to write down dates, times, and names of who you spoke with at the billing office. Follow up with the insurance carrier to make sure that a corrected claim/bill was sent to them.

KEY TERMS:

Codes

A set of numbers, letters, or a combination of both that describes a patient's procedure, service, supplies, medicine, durable medical equipment, and diagnoses.

Current Procedure Code (CPT)

A code describing a service or procedure. Located on the EOB and the bill.

Duplicate Charges

Charges billed multiple times to a patient for the same service.

Diagnosis (DX) Code

A code used to describe the patient's condition. Located on the claim and not the patient's bill in most cases.

Explanation of Benefits (EOB)

Sent to the patient by the insurance company to explain what charges were billed to them and how they were processed.

3

DID YOU OVERPAY?

Jason, twenty-two, went in for an eye exam. He was asked to pay his out-of-pocket expenses up front prior to this service being rendered. The payment consisted of a copay and coinsurance amount. Jason's provider billed the insurance company. After the insurance carrier processed the claim, the EOB stated that Jason owed less than what he paid up front. Therefore, Jason overpaid. The billing doctor may not necessarily inform Jason of his outstanding credit.

What should Jason do now? Has this ever happened to you? Have you wondered how to get the credit returned to you?

Like Jason, you should match your EOB with the bill that you received from your healthcare provider. Make sure that the bill correlates with your EOB. Again, pay attention to the following: the amount billed, amount not covered, deductible amount, copay amount, coinsurance amount, discount/contractual adjustment amount, and patient responsibility.

Once you have reviewed everything, make sure you pay only what you are responsible for per your explanation of benefits.

After the doctor's office has confirmed that he did overpay, Jason should request his refund. Not every Jason knows to call. And, once he's called and his refund has been processed, he (and you!) should ask, "By the way, do I have any other credits on my account?"

Refunds are no joke. They don't need to stay hidden. They don't need to grow interest in the wrong account. If you don't call, the refund creates a credit. This is your cash in your doctor's stash.

Overpayments Are Your Cash in Your Doctor's Stash

There are millions of dollars sitting on provider's books, aka the doctor's stash, that are due back to patients and/or insurance companies. There have been instances when patients have made payments based on the bill they received; however, their insurance company/EOB stated that they owed less than what they were being billed for. A credit is a credit whether it is an overpayment paid before the service or paid after the service. Either way, the patient needs to call the doctor's office and ask for a refund. The EOB is the evidence for the refund request.

Hospital Vs. Primary Care Provider (PCP)

Sometimes you have to decide if you're going to the hospital/emergency room or if you are going to schedule an appointment to see your PCP. Keep in mind that sometimes you don't have a choice.

Going to a hospital or PCP will determine how many bills you might receive, which will ultimately affect your out-of-pocket expense. If you go to a hospital facility, you may receive multiple bills, which means you will likely be paying more. This could consist of a bill from the hospital, treating doctor(s), radiologist, lab, etc. If you are going to see your PCP, you will likely only receive one bill.

24

Trish went to the emergency room because she was having stomach pain. She was seen by the emergency room (ER) doctor, who put in an order for a scan of her belly. She was taken to radiology for the scan and then brought back to the treatment area. The ER doctor came back to see Trish in the treatment room and advised her that everything looked fine. The ER doctor recommended that she follow up with a gastrologist (stomach doctor), and she was discharged to go home.

Trisha received multiple bills for her visit to the emergency room. She received bills from the hospital, the ER doctor, and the radiologist.

Do I Have a Credit On My Account?

This is the question that should be asked every time a patient visits the doctor, and/or if you are speaking with them. If the credit is not requested or claimed, the credit sits in the doctor's, facility's, or organization's account and grows interest. This is cash that could be used to take care of a patient's other medical bills or other financial responsibilities. Imagine being able to use those credits toward a vacation. Yes, a vacation! Sometimes credits are so significant that they can be used for other costly expenses or financial needs and wants.

Did I Keep Track of Who and What Amount Was Paid?

Once payments are made by the insurance carrier or another party on the patient's behalf for the service rendered, contact the provider initially paid and ask them if there is a credit on the account. If there is a credit balance, request that the provider send the refund or apply it to existing or future patient services.

Providers may hold on to the refund if there are charges pending on the account to be processed by the health insurance carrier or other parties, or if you have outstanding self-pay balances due. Follow up after two weeks to see if the charges pending have been processed. Keep in mind that you are well within your right to ask for a refund as many times as you see fit.

Was the Correct Provider Paid?

Each service and/or procedure can generate multiple bills/claims from different providers, hospitals, or labs. If you have insurance, and your deductible has not been met, then the deductible payment made per the request of the provider (the payment you made at registration before the service was rendered) will be applied to the first processed claim received by the insurance carrier.

Sometimes the provider name creates confusion. For example, you might receive a bill from Abraham Lincoln Hospital, and you might receive a bill from Abraham Lincoln Medical Associates. The hospital bill would be for the equipment used, and the Medical Associates bill would be for the doctor who actually treated the patients or read the results. Patients sometimes pay one provider but actually meant to pay another. Or, they thought the bill they paid was for the entire service received.

It can be challenging to get money back from any provider if paid in error, especially if outstanding balances currently exist on an account.

Consider reviewing each bill at least twice. Once by yourself, and then with a friend. Sometimes your emotional connection to a procedure interrupts your ability to understand the bill. A friend can offer you some clarity. Ask yourself, or have your friend ask, the following questions:

1. Who should payment be made payable to?

2. Are you paying the provider, facility, or lab?

3. What is the amount due?

4. How should payments be made (online or mailed to an address)?

5. Where should payments be sent (if mailing)? Remember to match the address on the bill.

Did the Insurance Company Pay After You Paid?

Patients pay up front for services in full or make a payment because they receive a bill or were asked to prepay. Some patients may make payments before their health insurance company or a third-party payer (such as a workers' compensation carrier, travel insurance, auto insurance, etc.) pays the provider. And/or the insurance company can also make a payment based on the patient's plan for the services rendered by the provider. As a result, three or four different parties have attended to the same bill. This causes a credit on the patient's account due to an overpayment, which puts more cash in the doctor's stash. You may never know the insurance paid after you, unless you call and ask the provider or insurance company, or review your EOB.

If the overpayment is due back to the patient, health insurance carrier, or third party, it will require a refund request. However, providers are not so quick to give refunds back to patients or insurance companies unless the patient or the insurance company initiates the request. If the patient wants their money back, they must do their due diligence and initiate the request first, and, in a lot cases, follow up throughout the process until they receive the actual refund. Providers *should* keep track and notify patients, insurance carriers, and other parties of overpayments received. In a perfect medical billing office world, this would happen. However, the reality is not that perfect.

Was a Traceable Method of Payment Used?

Patients sometimes pay for services with cash, in which case the transaction does not get recorded. Always ask for a receipt of payment and avoid paying a healthcare provider with cash. If a payment is made with cash and the receipt gets lost, the payment may not be traceable. For example, if the provider's billing staff did not post the payment, or they posted it to an incorrect account, and/or they cannot locate your payment, it will be difficult to trace the cash payment without the receipt. It will be difficult to prove that the payment was made.

Always pay with a traceable payment method. These methods include checks, debit cards, credit cards, or money orders.

If paying with a money order, make a copy of the front and back of the full money order. Should the money order copy get lost, it will be difficult to provide proof of payment to the provider's billing office. Remember to file the copy of the money order in a familiar place.

TAKEAWAYS:

- Always obtain a receipt when making a payment.
- Keeping track of what and who has been paid is extremely important.
- If a receipt from the provider is not obtained at the time of payment, it may be difficult to substantiate proof of payment, especially if paid in cash.
- Pay with a traceable method.

KEY TERMS:

Doctor's Charges

Services rendered to a patient from the provider.

Facility/Hospital Charges

Where services were rendered. (Usually the hospital or a facility that is not owned by a doctor.)

Overpayment

Payment made in excess of what is or was due.

NOTES

4

DO YOU HAVE MULTIPLE CARRIERS?

John, twenty, a second-year college student, was feeling under the weather and went to see his healthcare provider. Although he had primary and secondary insurance carriers, John only provided the provider's office with his primary provider's information. John later received a billing statement from his provider's billing office that showed he owed a balance after the primary insurance had paid. Confused, John called the provider's billing department to inquire about the remaining balance. The billing representative explained that his primary insurance carrier paid a portion of his bill and that he was financially responsible for the remaining balance.

John was concerned about his credit being negatively impacted and contacted his parents for advice on his patient responsibility. His mom asked him if he provided his secondary insurance information to his provider; he then realized that he had not. He contacted the billing office the next day and shared that he had another insurance company that he wanted them to bill. The information was updated and billed to the carrier. In 21 days, John received an updated billing statement from his provider, showing that the remaining balance was paid in full, and he did not owe anything. If he had not called back within thirty to sixty days (or the particular timely filing limit set by your insurance company) to share his secondary insurance carrier, he would have been responsible for the remaining balance.

Because John provided this information within the approved specified time frame after services were rendered, the provider was able to bill the secondary insurance carrier for the remaining balance. Had he not provided this information within the approved time frame after services were rendered, the provider would not have been able to bill the secondary insurance carrier, and he would have been financially responsible for the balance.

Before you go in for that appointment, make sure you know which insurance plan or plans you are currently enrolled in. Especially if you are a college student who has no clue how an unpaid medical bill can haunt and destroy your credit. That is the last thing you want to realize when you are trying to establish a career, family, or even want to purchase a home after graduation.

When a patient has multiple insurance carriers, there are specific claim guidelines that must be followed by the billing department. These are set by the insurance carrier. An example of having multiple carriers is when a patient is covered under their employer's plan and their spouse's plan. Another example would be a child covered under their parent's plan or even additionally a stepparent's plan. Knowing how many insurance carriers a patient has is important because each carrier should be billed. If all insurance carriers are not disclosed to the provider, and a claim is billed to only one of the carriers, the patient could possibly be held liable for part of or the entire bill. Providing all insurance carrier information is important so that patient responsibility will be minimal to none.

Most patients are aware if they have more than one insurance plan. For some reason, they may tend to think one plan may be better than the other. In some cases, one plan might offer more coverage, but it is to your benefit to share all the insurance carriers at the same time, in order for your claim to be processed correctly. There are certain factors based on carrier guidelines that determine which carrier would be considered primary, secondary, or even tertiary. One factor is the birthday rule, which sets up the primary insurance with the guardian/parent whose birthday month comes first. Another factor is connected to the number of employees when weighing Medicare above or below an additional insurance. In addition, if the patient has multiple insurances, and Medicaid is one of them, Medicaid will always be the last carrier to be billed.

Regardless of whether you visit a doctor's office, a lab, urgent care, or a hospital, remember to provide all insurance information each time. Don't assume that one facility will share your insurance information with another provider, even if you see multiple providers (i.e., radiologist and physician) in the same facility, and/or even if you visit multiple places (i.e., the lab and doctor's office) on the same day. Providing all of your insurance information *at each visit* will help ensure that your responsibility for the remaining balance is minimum to zero.

TAKEAWAYS:

- Make sure you provide all insurance information to your provider and not just one carrier because you think one is better than the other.
- The information must be provided before the past timely deadline, or the provider may hold you liable.

KEY TERMS:

Timely Filing

A time limit in which the provider or patient has to submit a claim or requested information to the health insurance carrier

Primary Insurance

The insurance carrier to pay the claim first.

Secondary Insurance

The insurance carrier to pay the claim second.

Tertiary Insurance

The insurance carrier to pay the claim after the secondary.

5

DO YOU KNOW THE DIFFERENCE BETWEEN MEDI-CARE AND MEDICAID?

Martha, seventy-three, sharp in her thinking and very diligent about her bills, lives at home and is raising her teenage granddaughter. She found herself going in to see her doctor weekly. Due to Martha's age, she was covered under Medicare Part A and Part B. During Medicare's open enrollment, Martha decided to opt into a Medicare Advantage Plan. At one of her weekly visits, Martha told her provider's front desk staff that she had two insurance carriers—Medicare and Aetna Medicare Advantage—and requested that they update this information on her account.

The following month, Martha received a bill for one of her visits. She immediately called the billing office and inquired if her secondary insurance was billed. The front desk staff member that answered her call reviewed her account and advised her that she only had one insurance, the Medicare Advantage Plan, and that the front desk staff member who took her information at the time should have clarified this detail for her. Martha explained that she was also covered under Medicare Part A and Part B. The agent further explained to Martha that when you are eligible for Medicare and then decide to opt into an Advantage Plan, it takes the place of the traditional Medicare Plan. This means that you only have one insurance and not two different ones. Martha shared that she did not know this and thanked the agent for explaining it to her and stated that she would follow up with Medicare for detailed information and an understanding of her plan.

Medicare and Medicare Advantage Are Not the Same

Are you aware that Medicare and Medicare Advantage are not the same? When a patient has a traditional Medicare plan, that means they have Medicare Part A and Part B. When a patient opts into a Medicare Advantage Plan, this means that the traditional coverage no longer will process their claims, and that they will now be processed under the Advantage plan. The patient has the option to select either traditional Medicare, or the Medicare Advantage Plan. Please note that the patient will not have both.

Some providers' billing staff get confused with this difference, and that is why it is vitally important that you understand your benefits. Don't assume that every front desk staff member understands the details of all insurance plans.

Medicare is sponsored by the federal government. Coverage applies to individuals who meet the following criteria*:

- Age 65 or older
- Disabled individuals to include those under the age of 65
- ESRD (End-Stage Renal Disease)

- ALS (Lou Gehrig's disease)

*Go to Medicare.gov for more information on eligibility requirements and guidelines.

Medicare and Medicaid/HMO Are Not the Same

Thomas, thirty-eight, is a single dad who has been raising three boys alone since his wife died from a sudden illness. Currently, he is working for temporary agencies with no benefits. He decided to take night courses to become a certified IT programmer so he can get a permanent job with benefits. This new job could help him financially support the boys and ensure that they have health coverage.

Thomas applied for Medicaid insurance for himself and his boys at the social services office through his local state government. After the office reviewed his application, he was approved based on his household size and low income.

Medicaid is a federal and state government–issued insurance program. Patients typically pay $0 to a minimal copay. Coverage applies to individuals who meet the following criteria*:

- Income
- Household Size
- Pregnancy
- Elderly
- Disabled Individuals

*Go to Medicaid.gov for more information on eligibility requirements and guidelines.

Straight Medicaid will allow you to see any doctor who accepts Medicaid. However, after you are approved for it, most will need to opt into a Medicaid HMO Plan. After choosing the HMO Plan, you will only be able to see a provider that participates in that plan.

TAKEAWAYS:

- Sometimes patients get the "Medi" part of "Medicare" and "Medicaid" confused. Please be sure to look at your card and confirm which one you have when providing your information.
- Medicare and Medicare Advantage are not the same. Your claims will be processed by either one or the other.
- Medicare and Medicaid are not the same.
- Please understand that in most cases, once you are eligible for Medicaid, you will need to select an HMO.

KEY TERMS:

Traditional Medicare

An insurance program sponsored by the federal government. It is a trust fund that helps to pay the medical costs for those who qualify.

Medicare Advantage

Plans that are offered by private insurance companies and offer Medicare Part A and Part B benefits.

Medicaid

A federal and state government-issued insurance. It helps with the medical costs for people with limited resources and income, and those who qualify.

Medicaid Health Maintenance Organization (HMO)

Medicaid HMO is a Health Maintenance Organization plan. Patients are only able to see providers within that network.

NOTES

6

PAY LESS FOR MEDICAL EXPENSES BEFORE AND AFTER SERVICE

The billing system is complex, and it is not unusual for you to get a bill for a payment you do not owe.

While walking down the stairs to do laundry, Gina tripped and slid down ten steps. She began to feel pain in her back and noticed a slight discomfort in her wrist. She called her PCP to make an appointment. The front desk staff told her to come in and that they would see her as soon as possible. They also advised her that her doctor was not available, but another doctor in the office was able to see her.

In order to ensure that Gina's out-of-pocket medical expenses are minimal, she would need to ask some important questions of both the insurance company and the new doctor before she decides to visit. Gina should share the information between the insurance company and her doctor's office in order to minimize errors. Gina should not assume that the front desk staff has all the correct answers.

How Do You Pay Less Before the Medical Expenses Are Incurred?

Questions to ask include:

1. Does this office take my insurance?
2. Does this office visit require a referral?
3. Is this doctor, facility, and/or provider in-network or out-of-network?
4. Will this be coded as an emergency or office visit?
5. Will I be asked to sign documents? What are they? What do the mean?
6. What are self-pay discounts? Does this office offer a self-pay discount if I don't have insurance?

Does the office take my insurance?

Some offices may accept and bill your insurance, but the doctors/ facility may not participate with your insurance. If they participate, you will pay less. If they do not participate, you will pay more.

Does this office visit require a referral?

You can find out if you need a referral by contacting your insurance company and the provider's office. If one is needed, you will need to obtain it from your PCP. Obtaining one will ensure that you pay less when receiving services from a specialist.

What is a referral?

A referral is a written order from a provider to see a specialist to receive certain specialized services. Although it is best practice for patients to obtain the referral and provide to the specialist or the provider may inform the patient that one is required by their insurance carrier, there is no law stating that the providers have to do so. Providers may obtain the referral for the patient because they want to make every effort to ensure that they receive timely reimbursement and are ensuring that the patient benefits guidelines are being addressed. This service also provides a good patient experience, which helps ensure patient retention.

Bring the referral.

Always be proactive and do your due diligence. Call the insurance company to let them know the service you anticipate having and ask if a referral is required. Do not depend on your healthcare provider to do this for you, even though they should. Some are very good at doing this, and some are not, meaning they can drop the ball. If a referral is required, make sure you obtain one from the necessary provider. Make a copy for your records and give the original to the provider at the time of your service or appointment.

Is the doctor and/or provider in-network or out-of-network?

The answer to this question will determine if a patient pays more or less. If the provider is in-network, the patient will pay less. If the provider is out-of-network, the patient will pay more. When the provider has a negotiated contract with the insurance company, they are considered in-network. When the provider does not have this negotiated contract, then they are considered out-of-network.

Will this be coded as an "emergency visit" or an "office visit"?

Patients should always ask a provider's office and/or urgent care facility if their charges will be billed as an emergency visit or office visit. Either location can answer this question better than the insurance company. The coding of your visit will determine if you will pay more or less based on your plan benefits.

What is this document I am being asked to sign?

If you are asked to sign the payment authorization form, the waiver form, and/or the Advanced Beneficiary notice form before services are rendered, remember to pause and ask questions. One question could be, "Will this document hold me completely responsible if the service is not covered by the insurance?" If you are unsure about what your insurance will or will not cover, you can choose not to sign the forms, but the facility can choose not to continue the service. The documents that you sign could potentially hold you completely financially liable for the service.

These are a lot of questions, and you might forget to ask all of them in an emergency. Even in a non-emergency, you may forget to ask. Don't worry; when you are in the waiting room, you can pull these questions out of your wallet or pocket and ask the front desk. But remember, they may or may not have all the answers. After the doctor's visit, I encourage you to call the insurance company and ask these questions if you forgot to do so before services were rendered.

What are self-pay discounts?

If you do not have insurance, this is the moment to ask about self-pay discounts. Sometimes this could be 10%–20% off of the total charge and requires the doctor's approval.

How Do You Pay Less on Medical Expenses After the Service Has Occurred?

Review the bill and the EOB and ask the following questions. You may have to pick up the phone and call both the insurance company and the provider for answers.

A) Was the correct insurance carrier billed?

B) Are these duplicate charges?

C) Did the insurance company pay my claim?

D) Was the claim processed in-network or out of network?

E) Was the claim processed without the referral?

F) How can I obtain the copy of the referral for the claim?

G) Is additional documentation required?

H) Were the adjustments applied?

I) Are there any credits on my account from previous overpayments that can be applied to my current outstanding balance?

Was the correct insurance carrier billed?

Check with the provider to make sure they billed the correct insurance. If you have more than one insurance, confirm that you have provided them all, and be sure to let the provider know the correct order in which they should be billed. Also, document the date that the provider sent the bill to the insurance company.

Are these duplicate charges?

Sometimes the provider will accidentally duplicate the same service twice on the same day. In other words, one office visit suddenly appears as two on the bill.

Did the insurance company pay my claim?

You may receive a bill before the insurance company has paid the claim. You should contact them prior to paying if you have not received your EOB to check the status of the claim processing.

Was the claim processed in-network or out-of-network?

Once you are seen by your provider and your charge has been billed to your insurance company and processed, review your EOB to verify that your claim was processed in-network, or out-of-network. If you are unsure, contact your insurance carrier and ask them. Sometimes health insurance carriers will process your claim out-of-network in error. Providers will not always catch this mistake, and they may accidently bill you for the out-of-network balance.

If it does happen, this will cause the provider to bill you for an amount that you do not owe (your cash, their stash). Instead, pause, breathe, and contact your provider and/or the insurance company to request that the claim be sent back for reprocessing. Your provider should advise you that they will follow up with the carrier and place that invoice on hold pending a response from the carrier.

Was the claim processed without the referral?

If you are unsure how to determine if your claim was processed with or without your referral by reviewing your EOB, call your insurance carrier directly and ask them for confirmation. You will need to provide them with the following:

- Your member ID
- Your name
- Your date of birth

- The date of service
- The total charge for the service billed by the provider or facility

Even if you do not have all of the information, the insurance carrier will still most likely be able to locate the claim in question.

Then, when you have verified that the claim was processed without the referral, you should follow these steps:

1. Contact your provider's billing office.

2. Request they send the referral to the insurance carrier and request that the claim be reprocessed.

3. Request that they put your bill on hold until they receive an updated response from your insurance company. Typically this takes between 14–30 days.

In some cases, the provider may not be able to locate your referral even though you gave it to them. If this occurs, provide them with a copy of your referral.

How can I obtain a copy of the referral for the claim?

Contact the referring provider to get a copy of the referral.

You can also contact your insurance carrier and let them know you have a copy that you can send to them for processing. If the insurance company allows you to send them a copy of the referral, obtain the following information:

- The fax number and/or email address
- A name or department to address the fax/email to
- The claim number and/or a reference number

Be sure to fax the referral to the insurance company with all of the information stated and keep a copy of the information and confirmation of the fax for your files.

Going to the Specialist

Remember to give the original referral to the provider. If you are going to send the copy of the referral that your PCP gave you to the specialist, obtain the following information:

- The fax number or email address
- A name or department to address the fax or email to

Information can get lost and conversations can be forgotten. It is important to keep documentation of all communication that you have with your provider, and/or the insurance carrier.

The referral makes a big difference. It will determine if you will pay more or less.

Is additional documentation required?

Once the insurance company receives and processes the medical claim, supporting documentation may be requested from the provider. If the information is not sent in a timely manner, the insurance company will complete the claim processing and notify the provider that it was denied. They will also notify the provider that they cannot bill the patient for the charge. In many instances, the provider may still inadvertently bill the patient for the denied claim amount/charge, and the patient is not responsible for the bill—a bill that the carrier has denied because the additional information has not been received.

In addition, the carrier may ask for additional information (i.e., accident details, prior records from another provider) from the patient, and if it is not received, the patient will be liable for the claim amount/charge. Pay attention to and read the EOB to determine why the insurance company did not pay the claim and to verify the patient's financial responsibility.

If necessary, contact the provider's billing office to advise them that you are aware of the claim denial because they did not send the requested information on time. Therefore, you are not financially responsible, and they need to apply an adjustment to (or "write off") the balance per your EOB. Put this request in writing with a copy of your EOB and send it to the provider via a traceable method, such as email, fax, or certified mail. It is best to send it at least two different ways.

Were the adjustments applied?

The EOB is sent to the patient by the insurance carrier, which explains if the insurance carrier applied any *adjustments* to the charges submitted by the healthcare provider.

But…

The EOP is sent to the healthcare provider by the insurance carrier and it explains how payments are processed. The patient will not receive the EOP but it is the same as the EOB, which the patient can request from the insurance if they have not already received it.

Compare the bill you received from the healthcare provider and/or the facility with your EOB. Pay close attention to the column that states *Contractual Adjustment* or *Adjustment*. Some adjustment verbiage may be slightly different based on the insurance carrier.

What is an adjustment?

An *adjustment* is an amount written off by the healthcare provider as a loss of income. Adjustments are not to be paid by the patient. Sometimes, providers or facilities still bill patients for adjustments after the insurance carrier advises them not to, which causes patients to make payments they are not responsible for.

Why does this happen?

Most often, billing patients for adjustment amounts is not intentional. Sometimes, the electronic file of the EOP from the insurance carrier does not post correctly to the patient's account information and the provider's billing system.

Also, the provider's accounts receivable department may not have posted the payments correctly based on the EOP.

Were you billed for the adjustments?

Every time you get a bill from a provider or facility, match it against your EOB.

Your EOB is a document that your health insurance carrier sends to you. This document has many important parts, and in regard to understanding adjustments, you should focus on these four categories:

- Total charges
- Payment amount
- Contractual adjustment
- Patient responsibility

The total charges include the amount that was received by the insurance carrier; the payment amount is the amount the insurance company paid to the provider; the contractual adjustment is the amount the insurance company tells the patient that they are not responsible for (this amount should be written off by the provider); and the patient responsibility is the amount that the patient is responsible for and should pay to the provider.

There are other adjustments you may need to confirm with your carrier if you or either the provider are responsible for, such as additional non-covered charges. Please note that some non-covered charges may or may not be your responsibility. A lot of factors can determine whether you are responsible.

Please check with your insurance company to verify if you are responsible for these amounts if they are reflected on your EOB.

I can't stress this enough: be careful and don't pay anything that is stated to be a contractual adjustment reflected on your EOB.

Here is an example of a woman who was billed for an adjustment that was not her responsibility:

Stephanie had a medical procedure performed by her provider at a hospital. When she received her bill, she noticed she was charged for an amount that was questionable, and it didn't match her EOB. Stephanie did not pay the provider's bill, and it was sent to collections. Inevitably, it was placed on her credit report as an unpaid collection account. Unfortunately, she did not understand that her EOB stated that this service should not be billed to her, or should have adjusted off because it was included in the hospital's bill. After Stephanie reviewed her EOB and consulted with her insurance carrier, she contacted her provider and requested that they apply the adjustment that was incorrectly billed to her and requested that the provider remove this from collection and update her credit report.

Are there any credits on my account from previous overpayments that can be applied to my current outstanding balance?

This question about a possible credit can and should be asked multiple times. It could be asked before you have a service, but it could be asked after you review your EOB and know exactly what you are financially responsible for. It could also be asked before you sign that check and put it in the mail. Do not assume that the front desk staff will automatically apply a past credit to an outstanding balance.

Financial Assistance/Charity Program

This is a program for individuals who cannot afford to pay their bills.

Each organization or provider has its own eligibility guidelines.

If you receive a bill and are financially indigent, ask the provider if they have either program. The key is to ask *before* your account goes to collections.

If a financial assistance program is available, request the application. Once you receive it, complete it and attach the requested/required documentation to it. You should then fax and/or email it to the provider's billing office. The information to be requested will likely include:

- Household size
- Proof of income
- Tax information
- Written statements
- Expenses.

Typically, if approved, the medical expense can be adjusted up to the full amount of the bill based on the poverty/provider's guidelines.

In conclusion, please remember, errors happen every day, especially when providers deal with a large volume of accounts. Some providers may not have enough staff to efficiently attend to each account with the level of detail needed.

Sometimes the provider's billing staff may not have complete knowledge or understanding of what is required by the patient or insurance company to bill both correctly.

If a provider confirms the patient's financial responsibility at the time of service and his or her cost share has not been met, then that provider may request to collect what will be owed prior to or at the time of services rendered.

It is well within your right to say, "Please bill me for it." Keep in mind that the provider can honor your request or decline it.

Finally, remember that financial aid does exist.

Providers and Hospitals provide financially indigent and qualified low-income patients with financial assistance. If approved for the assistance, patients receive free or reduced cost of care. For-profit providers (i.e., the doctors) are not obligated to honor such approval, even if the nonprofit hospital honors it.

Still, many other providers and facilities offer financial assistance. If you have a bill that you cannot pay, ask the provider if they have a financial assistance or charity program.

TAKEAWAYS:

- Did you know that unpaid medical bills can impact your credit?
- Did you know that you have the right to ask why you owe something?
- Did you check to see if the adjustment was applied?
- Did you know that providers will waive up to the full amount of your patient responsibility if you qualify?

KEY TERMS:

Adjustment

The patient is not responsible for this amount. It is a write off and loss to the provider

The patient can request an adjustment on the total bill, and/or the healthcare provider can offer this to the patient.

Duplicate Bill

A bill sent to a patient that was previously paid.

Explanation of Benefits (EOB)

The EOB is sent to the patient by the insurance company that explains what charges were billed to them and how they were processed.

Explanation of Payments (EOP)

An EOP is a payment remit sent to a healthcare provider from the insurance company explaining how the claim was processed.

Referral

Document/form referring the patient to see a specialist.

Financial Assistance

When the provider agrees to waive a portion or all of the patient's account balance based on their inability to pay criteria and guidelines.

In-Network Providers

Participating providers who have contract with a specified insurance plan.

Non-Covered Services

Non-covered services are charges that are not eligible for payment under the healthcare plan. Whether or not a patient is responsible for payment will depend on the healthcare plan coverage and/or if the provider has a waiver on file for the rendered service(s).

Out-of-Network Providers

Non-participating providers who do not contract with a specified insurance plan.

Self-Pay/Discounted Balance

A self-pay/discounted balance is a discount off of the original charge to a patient because they do not have health insurance, or the provider has agreed to give a discount on the service.

NOTES

7

HOW DOES COVID-19 IMPACT
YOUR MEDICAL BILLS?

Paula, sixty-five, woke up with a persistent dry cough and a loss of taste. Due to the current COVID outbreak, Paula decided to take her temperature. Surprisingly, her temperature registered 103°. Paula immediately drove to the nearest hospital. After checking in at the front desk, she provided her insurance information and received triage for her symptoms. The ER doctors decided that Paula would receive the test for COVID-19. She was discharged and advised she would be contacted in three days with the results. Seven days later, Paula received her results, and they were positive. Paula was asked to quarantine for fourteen days, and if symptoms worsened, to come back to the emergency room for further assessment.

Paula later received a bill from the emergency room visit. The facility requested a copay from her. After carefully reviewing the bill and being made aware of the federal guidelines related to cost-share waivers, Paula contacted her insurance carrier to question how her claim was processed. The insurance carrier advised her that the bill received from the provider did not have a COVID-related diagnosis. She contacted the providers billing office to advise them that she should not be responsible for any copay cost-share because the service was COVID-related and requested that they review the coding. After the coding was reviewed and updated, her claim was resubmitted to her health insurance carrier and reprocessed. The new bill sent to her reflected that her patient copay responsibility was zero.

Paula tested positive for COVID-19. She was lucky enough to recover. But many patients around the world have not survived. According to the CDC, as of June 4, 2020, there have been a total of 1,842,101 cases, and a rise of 800 new cases per day. In the United States alone over 107,029 people have died.

This pandemic doesn't create equality in medical care, and the cost varies state by state and even within some states. Some states have made testing free, while other states are charging for tests and Personal Protective Equipment (PPE).

Emergency rooms are flooded with patients, admissions are on the rise, and telemedicine appointments have become the new norm for providers and patients. It is important to remember that the healthcare system is struggling, and it will take time, resources, and restructuring to recoup.

If you are admitted to the hospital, make sure you provide the correct guarantor information. The guarantor is the person who will be responsible for the bill and interpretation. This person should also be ready to review all charges on the bill to ensure that they are accurate, that the charges were billed to the insurance carrier, or if the patient was deemed as a self-pay patient, that they are only being billed for the amount that they were quoted.

The White House has said there will be no surprise medical bills related to COVID-19. However, don't be surprised if you receive a medical bill. Now more than ever, it is important to understand your individual responsibility for copays, deductibles, and coinsurance.

As federal guidelines continue to evolve, most, if not all, insurance companies have adopted the federal government's position. All or most have waived copayments for COVID-19 testing and related visits. Some have even implemented patient cost-share waivers for coinsurance and deductibles for specified periods. Please review your individual healthcare plan's website for detailed information regarding their updated policies during this pandemic. Additionally, you can call your insurance company for clarification on their policies and procedures.

Some common errors on COVID-19 bills include:

- Duplicate charges
- Charges for services never received
- Incorrect charges
- Incorrect coding; if it is due to COVID-19, it needs to have a related code
- Being billed for a copay that should be waived due to COVID-19 insurance guidelines
- Insurance never billed
- Insurance company payments and adjustment not posted correctly

If you receive a bill in relation to a COVID-19 visit, you should review it thoroughly for the errors listed above. There have been many instances where patients have brought billing discrepancies to the provider's attention. When the charges have been researched and reviewed, patient disputes have in fact been accurate, and corrections were made to the bill.

Always remember you can ask for help to reduce your bill/patient responsibility. Please refer back to the second half of Chapter 6 and apply the "how to pay less" questions included to help you reduce your bill. And I am here to help you. Please consider emailing me at **info@ allaspectsmedical.com** if you need assistance.

Payment plans, courtesy adjustments, bill reductions, and financial assistance are available. You must, however, directly ask your provider's billing office about these options.

TAKEAWAYS:

- All or most payers have waived copayment for COVID-19 testing and visits for a specified period.
- Review your individual health plan's website.
- Don't be afraid to question about any bill that you receive.
- If you have been affected by COVID-19, call your insurance carrier to verify your individual cost share responsibility.

KEY TERMS:

COVID-19 Waiver

Cost share waiver per the insurance company related to current pandemic.

PPE

Personal protective equipment used by providers when treating patients.

8

WHAT SHOULD YOU REMEMBER WHEN USING A FLEXIBLE SPENDING ACCOUNT (FSA) CARD OR A HEALTH SAVINGS ACCOUNT (HSA) CARD?

Rachel, the director of a major auto dealership, attended several orthopedic appointments in January to correct an ongoing issue with foot pain. During these visits, she was asked to pay a copay, and for a foot boot that would not be covered by her insurance. Rachel paid the requested amount with her Flexible Spending Account (FSA) card. Two weeks after she received her boot, she received a letter from her FSA card administrator requesting that she provide them with an itemized bill to verify that the charges that were processed were used for a qualified medical expense. Rachel contacted her provider and requested that they mail her an itemized bill. Once she received it, she mailed it to the FSA administrator.

Allyson, thirty-two, a high-school teacher, suffers from chronic pain in her body. She frequently visits many physicians every month to assist with the treatment of her condition. At the beginning of open enrollment for insurance with her employer, she chose a less expensive plan with a high deductible of $6,000. Allyson decided to opt into a Health Savings Account (HSA) plan, which would allow her to put pre-tax money into an account that could be used for medical, dental, vision, deductibles, and other medical expenses. Due to her condition, it was necessary for her to undergo an immediate procedure that required that she pay part of her deductible upfront. Allyson used her HSA card to take care of that payment and was able to take care of her bill prior to her procedure without worry.

Some companies provide their employees with the choice of either an FSA or an HSA, or both. Do you know if you have selected either of these options? And if you do have them, do you know that you must remember to request an itemized bill to submit to the account administrator?

Required Documentation

The FSA/HSA account administrator wants an itemized bill but may say the word "receipt" instead. Be sure to request the correct document from the provider. Often, patients will call and request a receipt, when in fact, they should request an itemized bill. An itemized bill provides detailed information needed by the FSA/HSA administrator to justify the use of the benefit card. The itemized bill includes:

- Date of service
- Coding (description of services)
- Charge amount
- Payments received

- Patient responsibility

An itemized bill also shows the FSA/HSA holder that the payment made went against a healthcare service during the specified timeframe covered.

If the itemized bill does not contain the required information, the card administrator, potentially, could deny the payment. The patient may incur a charge back to the FSA/HSA account, or they may not issue the benefit payment to the patient and/or put a hold on the card.

Upon receiving the itemized bill, make a copy for your records and email, mail, or fax the original to the FSA/HSA carrier.

Use It or Lose It

During the open enrollment period, choose carefully the exact amount of pre-tax dollars that you want to place on one or both cards because both plans could have a "use it or lose it" or "rollover" clause. That means if the funds in the account are not used within the benefit period, the funds will be lost and unavailable to the participant in some cases. Every employer has a different policy regarding their FSA or HSA. Contact your employer for availability, eligibility, and requirements.

HSA accounts can rollover to the next year, and in some cases, you can even use an accumulated specified amount to invest in a 401K for medical expenses. Check with your employer and/or a tax professional for more details.

TAKEAWAYS:

- Use your FSA benefits within the specified time period or you could possibly lose them.
- Request an itemized bill instead of a receipt to submit to the account administrator.
- Always keep a copy of the receipt and itemized bill for your records.

KEY TERMS:

Flexible Spending Account (FSA)

An account in which pre-tax dollars are deposited per pay period and used to pay for childcare or medical expenses not covered by an insurance carrier, such as copays, coinsurance, deductibles, and prescriptions.

Health Savings Account (HSA)

A savings account in which pre-tax dollars are deposited per pay period and used to pay for healthcare expenses such as high deductibles.

Itemized Bill

An itemized statement of charges for any service and services rendered to a patient. It may include total charges, payments, adjustment, and some procedure and diagnoses code information.

9

GET YOUR CASH FROM YOUR DOCTOR'S STASH

The two most important ways to get your cash include reviewing your EOB and calling the doctor's/provider's office. But remember that the doctor's office may also be communicating with insurance companies and vendors in order to gather important information regarding the services you received. All of this will assist you in account resolution and getting your cash. It is vitally important to document the names of who you spoke with and what you were told.

While taking notes regarding the nature of the conversation, be sure to obtain the following:

- Who?
- What?
- What office?
- What date/time?

- Get a name! Get a name! Get a name!

- Call reference number?

When you remember to document, these notes will assist you, the front desk, and billing staff in those situations where communication occurs among health care entities, and there has been little to no documentation of those on your account.

Calling the Doctor's Office

When you call the doctor's office, a customer service representative answers, and you introduce yourself while providing them with your account information. You then proceed to tell the representative your issue and/or concern. After researching your account, the agent discovers that there may be one or more things that need to be done on your account. These can include:

- Updating your account information

- Billing your insurance company

- Sending your account to another department for review

- Updating your address so that you will get a bill

- Escalating your inquiry to management

- Contacting the collection agency to update or close your account

After your call with the agent, they assured you that your inquiry would be addressed or processed. About a month later, you receive another bill and notice that the same issue is reflected on the billing statement.

You may ask why, when you were assured that your inquiry thirty days prior would be taken care of. There are many reasons that your issue may not have been resolved. They include:

- The agent did not do what they promised.

- The person or department that your inquiry was sent to never even reviewed the request.

- Your request was reviewed but not resolved, and it's either sitting on someone's desk or in a queue to be worked on.

- Your inquiry was lost, and it is not in transit to be resolved.

- Your inquiry was received and not addressed.

You would be surprised by how often information and communications between patients and the provider's clinical and billing staff get lost, or are said to have never happened.

What really ensures that your inquiry is resolved is if the representative did what they said they would do. If you are not sure, then contact the doctor's office or medical facility.

Document, Document, Document

Always write down the date, time, and name of the person spoken to. File this information for later reference if needed to expedite future requests. Once you have confirmed that the billing office has addressed your previous issue, and your inquiry has been completed, then ask the following questions:

- Are there any past self-pay balances on my account?

- Are there any past credits on my account that can be applied to the self-pay balance or balance owed after insurance paid the claim?

If yes, ask them for the refund of the credit on the account or apply to a outstanding self-pay balance. This is part one of your cash in the doctor's stash. It has lived there too long.

Secondly, since you have reviewed your EOB against the most recent bill, you have noticed that there is a new credit due back to you due to payment that you made. Request your refund. This is part two of your cash that just arrived in your doctor's stash.

Typically, refunds are sent in the form of a check or refunded back to the credit card used. Be sure to confirm the following:

- The address where you want the check to be sent

- The name the check will be made out to

- The estimated time it will take to process the check and when to expect it

If you get a hunch that something may not have been billed correctly, or you were overcharged and paid for something that your insurance company said you were not responsible for, you need to pick up the phone and call your provider's billing office. Even if you are nervous about asking questions, it is essential to do so in order to get your money back. I can't stress this enough; your money is growing interest. Don't forget to ask about past credits as well as current credits regarding your most recent doctor's visits.

TAKEAWAYS:

- Don't let your money sit there! Pick up the phone and request your refund.
- Getting the name of the person you spoke to and a date and time of when you spoke to them will be helpful when you're following up on an issue.

KEY TERM:

Interest

A percentage calculated off of a dollar amount.

NOTES

APPENDIX 1

TIPS TO HELP YOU GET YOUR MONEY BACK

There may be a credit sitting on your account, money that is due back to you from your healthcare provider.

Here are a few tips for what to do when reviewing the EOB:

- Read your EOB in its entirety before you pay the bill.

- Check the *patient responsibility section* and the *adjustment section* on the EOB. Those two areas will let the patient know what their specific responsibility is.

- Review the rejection code within the details of the processed information and compare it to the code and explanation on the bottom of the EOB. Take note of these details to use for future conversations with the healthcare provider and the insurance company.

Here are a few tips for what to do when reviewing the bill:

- Never assume the bill you receive from the healthcare provider is correct.

- Make sure that the bill you are paying to your healthcare provider is not a duplicate. Ask yourself, "Did I already pay this?"

- Review the charges on your bill to ensure that the service listed is correct.

- Make sure that the charges are not listed more than once (duplicate charges).

- Review the bill to make sure it belongs to you. Make sure that the patient's name, date of birth, address, and phone number are all correct. Make sure that the services stated align with the services delivered.

- If a year or more has passed, and you receive a bill for past services from a medical provider, you have the right to dispute the bill for untimely billing. The fact that they took a year to enter the services is one of many problems and/or a reason to dispute it requesting an adjustment.

Here are a few tips for talking with the healthcare provider:

Please ensure you provide all insurance information to your healthcare provider. This is especially true if you have more than one insurance carrier.

- Provide your correct insurance information to your healthcare provider, and confirm that they have the correct information at each visit.

- Call your healthcare provider and ask, "Do I have any credits on my account that are due back to me?" If they say yes, ask them to mail it to you directly, or to transfer it to an outstanding balance you may have.

- If you have noticed that your account went to collections, you can request that your bill be pulled out of collections due to an error the provider caused.

- Don't assume that they did what you asked them to do. Follow up with the provider in seven days. For example, you can ask: "Was the original conversation documented on the account?" "Was the itemized bill mailed?" "Was the insurance information updated?" "Was the balance adjusted off?"

Here are a few tips for talking with the insurance provider:

- You should receive an EOB for every claim processed by your insurance carrier. If you have not received your EOB, call your insurance carrier and ask, "Did you ever receive and process this claim?"

- Call your insurance carrier and verify if any referrals are needed for a service before the service is rendered, and obtain an original referral. Keep a copy for your records and provide the healthcare provider with the original.

- Check with your insurance carrier before a service is rendered to verify that the provider/facility is participating with your insurance. The provider or the insurance company may not participate (i.e., out of network), and if they do not, it will impact your out-of-pocket expense. Also, ask if your plan has tier levels, and if so, ask them to explain the levels.

- Make sure to ask the name of the customer service agent/front desk staff you spoke to. Make sure you also note the time and date you spoke to them along with noting the number you called, and/or any reference number associated with the call.

- Your claim could have been processed out-of-network, and it should have been processed in-network. Call your insurance to verify that your claim was processed under the correct benefit level.

Here are a few tips for the best method of payment:

- Pay with a traceable method and keep detailed records, such as the invoice number, check number, the amount that was paid, and to whom you paid it to.

- Read the fine print of everything you sign. The fine print is what could hold you liable for the bill. Waivers specifically state that you understand that the service is not covered, and you are financially responsible.

- Always request a receipt after making any payment to a healthcare provider or facility and keep it for your records.

- If you do not have insurance, ask the healthcare provider/ facility about self-pay discounts, prompt payment discounts, payment plans, charity, or financial assistance programs.

Here are a few tips related to Medicare and Medicare Advantage:

- Medicare Part A and Medicare Part B are not the same.

- Always review your Medicare card to verify your coverage effective dates for Part A and Part B.

- Medicare Part A covers hospital charges only, and Medicare Part B covers physician charges only.

74

- Medicare and Medicaid are not the same.

- Medicare and Medicare Advantage are not the same.

- You no longer have traditional Medicare when you opt into a Medicare Advantage plan.

Here are a few tips related to Medicaid and Medicaid HMO:

- If you have Medicaid or Medicaid HMO, you will typically have little to no patient responsibility.
- Medicaid will always be second to pay if you have other insurance.
- Verify if you have Medicaid or Medicaid HMO. Always verify eligibility dates for each carrier and provide those dates to your healthcare provider. This is very important for time claim processing and provider reimbursement.

APPENDIX 2

KEY TERMS

Additional Documentation

Information that the insurance company will request from the provider and/or the patient.

Adjustment

The patient can request an adjustment on the total bill, and/or the healthcare provider can offer this to the patient. This is an amount that is written off and is a loss to the provider.

Authorization Number

A unique number provided by the insurance carrier in order to receive payment for services.

Charity Care

When the provider agrees to waive a portion or all of the patient's account balance based on specific criteria and guidelines.

Claim/Claim Form

A unified billing form used to submit charges and services to healthcare insurance carriers.

Claim Number

A unique number assigned by the insurance company to a claim for charges that they received.

Codes

A set of numbers, letters, or a combination of both that describes a patient's procedure, service, supplies, medicine, diagnoses, and durable medical equipment.

Coinsurance

An out-of-pocket expense; a percentage of the cost for the service that was rendered to the patient. Percentages can start from 10, 20, 30 percent, or more. For example, if the coinsurance amount is 10% and the cost of service is $1,000, the patient's payment responsibility is $100.

Contractual Adjustment

Part of the charge amount that is negotiated by the insurance company and provider to be written off.

Copay

A flat fee paid for certain covered services, such as doctor visits, emergency room visits, prescriptions, or in-patient visits.

Current Procedure Code (CPT)

A code describing a service or procedure.

Deductible

An amount required to be paid by the patient each year before the healthcare plan starts paying benefits.

Demographic Information

The patient's name, date of birth, address, and phone number.

Diagnosis (DX) Code

A code used to describe the patient's condition.

Doctor's Charges

Services rendered to a patient from the provider.

Doctor's Stash

Overpayments remitted to providers from insurance companies, patients, and other parties that sit in their bank account or on their books and collect interest.

Duplicate Bill

A bill sent to a patient that was previously paid.

Duplicate Charges

Charges billed to a patient for the same service multiple times.

Explanation of Benefits (EOB)

The Explanation of Benefits (EOB) is sent to the patient by the insurance company to explain what charges were billed to them and how they were processed.

Explanation of Payments (EOP)

A payment remit sent to a healthcare provider from the insurance company explaining how the claim was processed.

Facility

Where services were rendered. (Usually the hospital, or a facility that is not owned by a doctor.)

Financial Assistance

When the provider agrees to waive a portion or all of the patient's account balance based on specific criteria and guidelines.

Flexible Spending Account Administrator

A company that works with your employer to ensure that you are using the Flexible Spending Account money for qualified medical expenses.

Flexible Spending

Money set aside by your employer from your salary tax-free that can be used for qualified medical expenses.

Guarantor

The person who is financially responsible for the patient's bill. The billing statement/EOB will always be sent to this person, even if the patient is an adult.

HIPAA-Health Insurance Portability and Accountability Act (1996)

A law that protects a patient's privacy rights regarding their PHI-Private Health Information.

In-Network Providers

Participating providers who have a contract with a specified insurance plan.

Insurance Credit

Money due back to the insurance carrier as a result of overpayment.

Insurance Refund

Money due back to the insurance carrier as a result of overpayment.

Interest

A percentage calculated off of a dollar amount.

Itemized Bill

An itemized statement of charges for any service rendered to a patient.

Itemized Statement

An itemized statement of charges for any service rendered to a patient.

Medicaid

A federal and state government-issued insurance. It helps with the medical costs for people with limited resources and income who meet the specific qualifications.

Medicaid HMO

Health Maintenance Organization Plan. Patients are limited to see only the providers within that network.

Medicare

A federal insurance program sponsored by the government. It is a fund that helps pay the medical cost for those who qualify.

Medicare Advantage

Plans that are offered by private insurance companies and offer Medicare Part A and Part B benefits.

Non-Covered Service

Service that the patient or guarantor may be financially responsible for because it is not covered by the insurance.

Out-of-Network Providers

Non-participating providers who do not contract with a specified insurance plan.

Out-of-Pocket Expense

The patient's responsibility, which can include a copayment, coinsurance, deductible, and/or non-covered service.

Overpayment

Payment made in excess of what is or what was due.

Past Timely Filing

Claim was not filed in a timely manner per the insurance carrier's guidelines.

Patient Credit

Money due back to the patient due to overpayment.

Patient Refund

Money due back to the patient due to overpayment.

Patient Responsibility

The amount that a patient is responsible for paying.

Primary Insurance

The carrier that will pay the claim first.

Provider

A physician, hospital, lab, or facility.

Referral

Document/form referring the patient to see a specialist.

Self-Pay

The patient does not have insurance and is responsible for the bill.

Self-Pay Balance

The amount that could result from a patient not having insurance, copay, coinsurance, deductible, or a non-covered service. This amount is billed to the patient.

Self-Pay Discount

An amount that is discounted off of the total charge when the patient does not have insurance.

Secondary Insurance

The insurance carrier that will pay the claim second.

Specialist

A provider who is trained in a specific field of medicine.

Supporting Documentation

Information that the insurance company will request from the provider and/or the patient.

Tertiary Insurance

The insurance carrier that will pay the claim after the secondary.

Traceable Payment Method

A credit card, check, money order, or debit card.

Traditional Medicare

Medicare is a federal insurance sponsored by the government. It is a trust fund that helps to pay the medical cost for those who qualify.

Waiver

A document that holds the patient financially responsible when signed for a non-covered service.

APPENDIX 3

TESTIMONIALS

1) I am writing to you to sing the praises of a most incredible employee in the Billing Office - Ms. Venus Senior, Customer Service Supervisor. Let me tell you how she successfully resolved my billing issue and got me my $749.69 overpayment after almost three months.

On April 1st, I was told by the Cosmetic Dermatology Dept. that I would be receiving a refund from the Billing Department for services that I prepaid for but could not be completed because my Doctor was leaving the CBA practice.

After waiting three weeks for my check, I started calling the Billing Office to determine when I would receive this refund. The Billing person I spoke with said the Dermatology department needed to contact them to verify services. She said she would contact them and get back to me. I never heard from her but called again and was told Dermatology didn't respond to billing... I myself called Dermatology many times and left messages asking them to speak with Billing, so I could get my overpayment but never received a reply. My Doctor, who left the practice, passed my message along to the Dermatology Supervisor. However, two and a half months later, I still had not heard anything and began to worry I would never receive my $749.69.

In mid-June and in despair, I called Billing again, and luckily for me Ms. Senior answered. Right away, I knew this was an employee who cared and would do everything she could to help me. She identified herself by FULL name, GAVE me her email address, and asked me to forward any emails I had received from the Dermatologist to her so she could work on my problem. She actually called me back when she said she would; she answered EVERY email I sent almost immediately and told me her work schedule so I would know when to contact her. She did not stop when Dermatology ignored her calls and emails and went right up the chain to Patient Services, keeping me informed all the way.

Almost three months later, and two weeks after Ms. Senior got involved, I received my full refund! I KNOW this would not have happened without her help because I had another billing issue in the past and never encountered such a dedicated employee who really wanted to help me resolve my issue.

I sincerely hope that Ms. Senior will be recognized and rewarded by CBA for her incredible problem-solving skills, her persistence, her dedication, and her wonderfully gentle and caring manner. She is a treasure! - Matt R.

2) I want to sing the praises of Venus Senior in billing. She finally resolved a seven-month problem with my getting bills [sic] for allergy shots even though I paid the copayment at the time of service, and CBA cashed my checks. Senior patiently spoke with me on the phone even though I was very upset, figured out what she needed from me,

provided me with her email address so that I could send her the needed documentation, and resolved the problem in ONE DAY. She followed up by phone and email to let me know that I now have a small credit on my account and sent me a bill showing a $0 balance due. She is my hero. I have been a patient at CBA since I moved to DC in 1979 and was insured through CBA's HMO until it closed. Since then, I made sure that CBA was part of my insurer's network, I was getting ready to find new doctors outside of CBA and am very happy that Ms. Senior was able to resolve the problem as I want to continue using CBA doctors. - Salina G.

3) For over six months, I have been trying to resolve a billing issue. It was only due to Ms. Venus Senior's Outstanding customer service that I did not give up hope and move to a different doctor. I was very frustrated, but Venus took time to listen to my side of the story, do the proper research, evaluate the facts, and help come up with a solution to my billing issue. Moreover, Venus followed up and called me to provide an update to my case. Venus persevered and solved my issue. I felt that she genuinely cared about my situation. I am grateful for the outstanding customer care she provided and hope she will be recognized. She is one of the most competent, sympathetic, and efficient customer service representatives I have over encountered. Thanks to Venus, you have a loyal CBA patient. - Kimberly C.

APPENDIX 4

IMPORTANT WEBSITES

Consumer Reports for Healthcare

https://www.consumerreports.org/healthcare-costs/prepay-hospital-bill/

NORC at the University of Chicago

https://www.norc.org/NewsEventsPublications/PressReleases/Pages/new-survey-reveals-57-percent-of-americans-have-been-surprised-by-a-medical-bill.aspx

Center for Disease Control (CDC)

https://www.cdc.gov/coronavirus/2019-ncov/cases-updates/cases-in-us.html

FINAL THOUGHTS

There are millions of dollars sitting in the doctor's stash. These millions of dollars belong to the insurance companies, patients, and even third-party payers at times.

It is important to make sure that you understand your benefits, EOB, and your patient responsibility.

Understanding will play a major part in making sure that your cash is not among the millions of dollars that are sitting and growing interest in an account that is not yours.

Keep records of the payments you make, every date of service, and the treatment you received, review your bill and EOB, call your insurance company, call the provider billing office, fax and email, and document who you speak to.

Lastly, don't let your cash sit and grow interest in their stash. Call today to inquire if you have a refund sitting out there due back to you.

Healthcare is a business that treats patients. Businesses are designed to make money. If it doesn't make money, it does not make sense.

Request your cash!

STAY CONNECTED WITH ME!

Website: www.allaspectsmedical.com

Email: info@allaspectsmedical.com or allaspectsmedical@gmail.com

Phone: 1-800-215-6708

 @allaspectsmedical
and Pay Less on Medical Expenses with "Venus"

 @allaspectsmedical

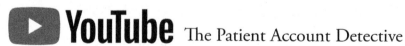 The Patient Account Detective

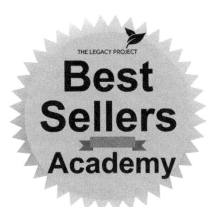

This book was published with the support of The Bestsellers Academy.

Do you have a book inside of you?

Let us get your story out of your belly and into an international bestselling book!

Phone: 1-868-374-7441

Email: success@thebestsellersacademy.com

Website: TheBestsellersAcademy.com

Made in the USA
Middletown, DE
15 September 2023

38402527R00056